Spanish Flu

The Story of the great influenza of 1918.

Gladys Maxwell

Contents

INTRODUCTION

The Spanish flu pandemic of 1918, has been recorded as the deadliest in history. It infected an estimate of 500 million people all over the world which was then, about one-third of the earth's population. When estimated, it was discovered that the disease killed about 20 million to 50 million victims, in which about 675,000 were Americans. The said Spanish flu was first discovered in Europe, the United States and then some parts of Asia before it's rapid spread all around the world. As at that time, there were no cure or effective drugs or vaccines that could treat this killer flu. The government of the various countries then, had to order it's citizens to wear masks. Public places such as schools, theaters and businesses were shut down and bodies of people who died from the flu were piled up in temporary morgues before the virus was wilted down.

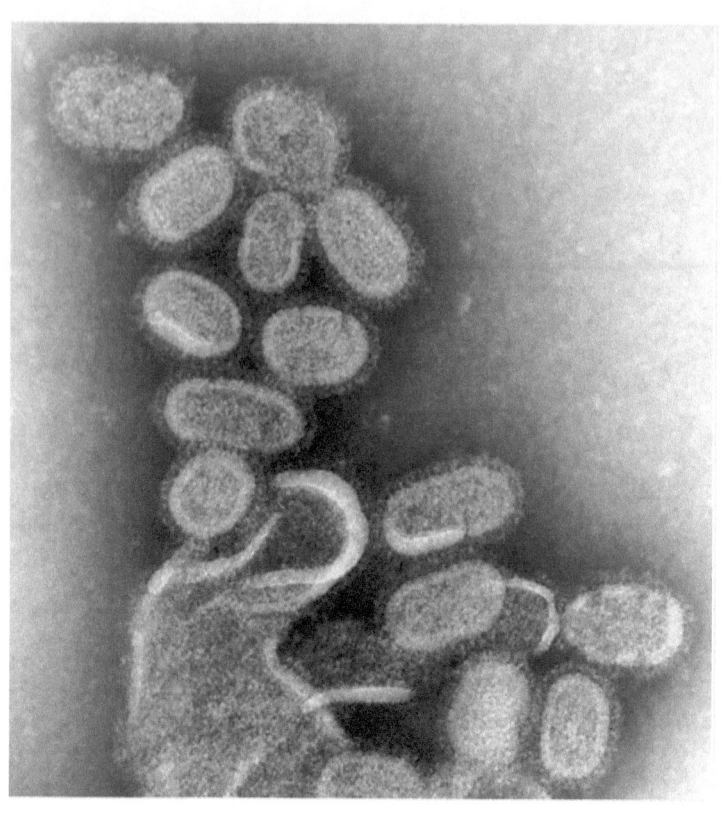

Chapter One: What is the flu?

Influenza, or flu as it is commonly called, is a virus which attack is on the respiratory system. This flu virus is highly contagious: If a person that is infected with the virus coughs, sneezes or talks, respiratory droplets will be generated and transmitted into the air. It can then be inhaled by anyone close by.

Also, anyone who touches something that has the virus on it and then goes on to touch his or her mouth, eyes or nose can become infected.

Flu Season

There are some seasons or weather conditions that are favorable for the flu to thrive. For example, in America the flu season is usually from late fall into spring. Sometimes in a year, more than 200,000 American citizens will be hospitalized because of complications and symptoms that are flu-related. And for over more than three decades past, there have been about 3,000 to 49,000 deaths caused by the flu in the U.S. in each year, recorded by the Centers for Disease Control and Prevention.

There is a particular category of people who face a higher risk of contacting the virus, they include: people that are above age 65, young children, pregnant women and people with specific medical conditions, e.g. asthma, diabetes or heart disease. These categories of persons mentioned above face a higher risk of getting flu-related complications, which includes pneumonia, ear and sinus infections and bronchitis.

A pandemic caused by a flu such as the one in 1918, usually happens when a virulent new influenza strain and for which little or no immunity appear. And such a flu spreads very fast rom person to person around the world.

Symptoms of the flu

The first time the flu appeared was in 1918. The pandemic happened in the spring of that year and was generally mild. Those who fell sick then will usually experience such typical flu symptoms like cold, fever and tiredness. They would recover normally after several days, and the number of reported deaths then was low.

But after a while, a second wave of highly contagious influenza appeared in the fall of that same year. Those who contacted it died just within hours or days of developing symptoms. Some of the symptoms include their skin turning blue and their lungs will get filled up with fluid which eventually causes them to suffocate. Just within the year 1918, the average life expectancy in the U.S reduced by a dozen years.

What Caused the Spanish Flu?

The actual cause of the flu is not exactly known. No one knew where the actual strain of influenza that caused the pandemic came from. However, the flu was first discovered in Europe, then America and some areas in Asia before it's rapid spread to almost every other part of the earth in just a few months.

Even though the 1918 flu was not isolated to one place, it became popularly known all around the world as the Spanish flu. The reason why it was regarded as such was because the disease hit Spain very hard and it was not subject to the wartime news blackouts which affected other European countries. (It was even reported then that Spain's king, Alfonso XIII, contracted the flu.)

One unusual thing that was noted about this flu of 1918 was that it affected and killed many people who were previously healthy, for example young people. People who were normally resistant to infectious disease such as this, including a number of World War I servicemen.

It was recorded that majority of the U.S. soldiers then died from the flu than the ones that were killed in battle during the war. It was also recorded that about

40 percent of the U.S. Navy was affected with the flu, while another 36 percent of the Army became very ill. And then the troops moving around the world inside crowded ships and trains also increased the rapid spread of the killer virus.

Although the death rate that was attributed to the Spanish flu is usually estimated to be around 20 million to 50 million victims all over the world. There were other estimates that was as high as 100 million victims which was then around 3 percent of the world's population. It is impossible to know the exact numbers due to lack of medical record-keeping in many places then.

What is however known is that there were few locations which was immune to the 1918 flu in the U.S. Some of the victims ranged from residents of most major cities to those of remote Alaskan communities. It was even reported then that President Woodrow Wilson contracted the flu just in the beginning of 1919 while he was still in the negotiating process of the Treaty of Versailles, which later resulted to the end of World War I.

Why Was the disease called The Spanish Flu?

It is important for you to know that the Spanish Flu did not originate in Spain, though news from the media made it seems so. During World War I. Spain actually was known to be a neutral country with a free media that covered information about the outbreak from the start. Spain reported the first outbreak of the flu when it was initially observed in Madrid in late May of 1918. But Allied countries and the Central Powers had wartime censors who covered up news about the flu to keep their morale high. So because Spain news sources were the only ones giving report about the flu, many people then believed it originated there. Whereas the Spanish believed the virus came from France and they called it the "French Flu."

Where Did the Spanish Flu Come From?

It is still not known even by scientists where the Spanish Flu originated from. Although there have been different stories speculating that the flu originated from France, China, Britain, or the United States. The first known case was reported in a camp known as Camp Funston in Fort Riley, Kansas City, on the 11th day of March 1918.

Some people even believe that infected soldiers spread the disease to other military camps across the country, and then brought it overseas. It is recorded in history that in March of 1918, 84,000 American soldiers headed across the Atlantic and were followed by another 118,000 the following month, so this gave rise to the believe that they were the ones who spread the flu overseas.

Chapter Two: Fighting the Spanish Flu

In 1918 when the flu started to hit very hard, doctors and scientists didn't know what to do, neither did they know what caused it or how to treat it. Unlike in these present times, there were no effective vaccines or antivirals, drugs then that could treat the flu. The first ever licensed flu vaccine came on board in America in the 1940s. When it got to the following decade, manufacturers of vaccine could now routinely produce vaccines that would help control and prevent future pandemics.

The complicated issue that arose then was the fact that World War I had left parts of America with a shortage of physicians and other health workers. And the few available medical personnel that were left in the U.S., came down with the flu themselves.

Also, some of the hospitals in most areas were so filled with flu patients that schools, people's private homes and other buildings had to be converted into temporary hospitals, s and some of these makeshift hospitals were staffed with medical students.

In some communities the officials there had to impose quarantines, ordered citizens to wear masks and shut down public places, including schools, churches and theaters. The government of the countries worldwide advised it's citizens to avoid shaking hands and to stay indoors. Libraries stopped lending books and regulations were passed banning spitting.

According to The New York Times, it was reported that during the pandemic, Boy Scouts in New York City would approach people that they had seen spitting on the street and give them cards that read: "You are in violation of the Sanitary Code."

Aspirin Poisoning and the Flu

As the situation got worse and no cure was found for the flu, a lot of doctors started to prescribe medication that they felt would reduce the symptoms. One of such prescription was aspirin, and aspirin had been trademarked by Bayer in 1899- a patent that expired in 1917, meaning new companies were able to produce the drug during the Spanish Flu epidemic.

Prior to when the hike in deaths got attributed to the Spanish Flu in 1918, the U.S. Surgeon General, Navy and the Journal of the American Medical Association had all recommended that aspirin be used for the flu. Even medical professionals advised patients to take up to 30 grams per day, a dose that is known now to be toxic and harmful. (As a need for comparison, the medical consensus today is that doses above four grams are not safe). Aspirin eventually caused its own damage, some of the symptoms of aspirin poisoning include hyperventilation and pulmonary edema. It also caused a buildup of fluid in the lungs, and it's now a belief that many of the October deaths were actually caused or aggravated by aspirin poisoning.

The Flu Takes Heavy Toll on Society

The flu was so bad that it was wiping out entire families, leaving many to become widows and orphans in its wake. Funeral parlors were overcrowded with bodies piled up. Most people had to dig graves by themselves for their own family members.

The flu also affected the economy a great deal. In the United States for instance, a lot of businesses were forced to shut down because so many employees contracted the flu and became sick. Even basic services like mail delivery and garbage collection could not be done because most of the workers were affected with the flu.

In some regions there weren't enough farm workers to harvest crops. Crops were thus left to wither, while people were in hunger. Most state and local health departments closed for business, thus affecting the efforts to reduce the spread of the 1918 flu and also affecting the provision of answers to the curious public.

How U.S. Cities Tried to Stop The 1918 Flu Pandemic

There was another wave of the Spanish flu that hit America shores in the summer of 1918 and this was quite devastating. This second wave came as a result of returning soldiers from states that were affected with the disease. They contacted it and brought it back thus making the flu to spread to the general population—especially in cities that was a bit crowded. Since there was no cure, vaccine nor an approved treatment plan, a burden fell on the local mayors and healthy officials to prepare alternative plans that will help to safeguard their citizens. Because many were faced with the pressure to appear patriotic at wartime and also having a censored media hiding the true rate of the disease's spread, most of them made tragic decisions.

Philadelphia took a slow approach in combating the flu. Dr. Wilmer Krusen, director of Public Health and

Charities for the city, insisted that the increasing fatalities were not a result of the "Spanish flu," but rather just the normal flu. With this report, the city on September 18, went forward to carry out a Liberty Loan parade in which tens of thousands of Philadelphians attended. And this made the disease to spread like wildfire, that just within the space of 10 days, more than 1,000 Philadelphians were dead, while another 200,000 fell sick. This was what led to then city closing down, schools, businesses and theaters. And by the time it got to March of 1919, more than 15,000 citizens of Philadelphia had died.

Unlike Philadelphia, St. Louis, Missouri, took a swifter approach in curtailing the flu. It's schools and movie theaters were closed down and public gatherings were banned. And because of this, the peak mortality rate in St. Louis was just about one-eighth of Philadelphia's death rate during the peak of the pandemic. The deaths due to the virus were estimated to be about 358 people per 100,000 in St Louis, compared to 748 per 100,000 in Philadelphia during the first six months—the deadliest period—of the pandemic.

In San Francisco, the citizens were fined $5, (which was a significant sum at the time) if they were caught in public places without having a mask on and such defaulting citizens would be charged with disturbing the peace.

Spanish Flu Pandemic Ends

By summer of 1919, the flu pandemic finally came to an end, because those that were infected with the flu either died or developed immunity.

After about 90 years later, precisely in 2008, some researchers announced that they had discovered what made the 1918 flu so deadly, this is their findings: That a group of three genes gave the virus the ability to weaken a victim's bronchial tubes and lungs and thus clearing the way for bacterial pneumonia.

After the 1918 flu, there have been several other influenza pandemics, although none has been as deadly as the Spanish flu. There was a flu pandemic from around 1957 to 1958 which killed about 2 million people worldwide, in which 70,000 of them were in the United States. Another pandemic also developed in 1968 to 1969 killed. This killed an estimate of 1 million people, including some 34,000 Americans.

Over 12,000 Americans died during the H1N1 (rather called "swine flu") pandemic which occurred from 2009 to 2010. Now, the novel coronavirus pandemic of 2020 is spreading swiftly around the world as countries are racing to find a cure for it and citizens have been advised to stay indoors in order to avoid spreading the disease. This is particularly deadly because many carriers of the disease do not show any symptoms for days before realizing they are infected.

This modern day pandemics is what brings renewed interest in and also attention to the Spanish Flu, or should I say "forgotten pandemic," because its spread was overshadowed by the deadliness of World War I and it was covered up by news blackouts and poor record-keeping.

The idea of Social distancing is not a modern idea. It was the strategy that was used to save thousands of American lives during the last great pandemic. Below is a description of how it worked.

The Spanish flu of 1918, lasted until 1920 and is still considered as the deadliest pandemic in modern history. Today, the world is working tirelessly to bring a halt to the recent pandemic that is spreading rapidly. Scientists and historians are carrying out researches and studying the 1918 outbreak just in case they can get clues to the most effective way to stop a global pandemic. The efforts implemented then to stop the spread of the flu in cities across America and the outcomes may possibly offer some lessons in battling today's crises.

Vast demographic changes in the past century have made it difficult to curtail a pandemic. Factors such as globalization, urbanization, and a larger, and more overpopulated cities can cause a virus to spread across a continent in a few hours. Meanwhile the tools available to respond have remained nearly the same (it has not been improved on). Just like in the past centuries, public health interventions are the first approach that will be used against an epidemic in the absence of a vaccine. And these measures include closing down schools, shops, restaurants e.t.c, it will also involve putting restrictions on transportation; mandating social distancing, and banning of public gatherings. (with this

smaller groups can save lives during a pandemic.)

But you know the difficult part is getting citizens to comply with such orders. For example, in 1918, a San Francisco health officer shot three people when one disobeyed the order to wear a mandatory face mask. Another example is Arizona, where a police officer handed out $10 fines for those caught without the protective gear. Eventually, these measures paid off. After a multitude of strict closures and controls on public gatherings was implemented, St. Louis, San

Francisco, Milwaukee, and Kansas City responded fastest and most effectively:

In 2007, there was a study in the Journal of the American Medical Association which did a critical analysis of the health data from the U.S. census that experienced the 1918 pandemic, and charted the death rates of 43 U.S. states. In that same year, two studies published in the Proceedings of the National Academy of Sciences made efforts to understand how responses influenced the disease's spread in different cities. Haven done a comparison of fatality rates, timing, and public health interventions, they discovered that death rates were about 50 percent lower in the cities that took preventative measures early on, as against those that did so late or not at all. The most effective efforts that had been taken so far is to close down schools, churches, and theaters, and also banning of public gatherings. This measure would allow time for researchers to come up with a possible vaccine (though in this 1918 case a flu vaccine was not used until the 1940s) that will lessen the strain on health care systems.

From the studies another important conclusion was reached: They observed that if the intervention measures are relaxed too early, it could make the situation to worsen. For example, St. Louis relaxed it's preventive measures early because of it's low death rate. They lifted the restrictions on public gatherings in less than two months after the outbreak started. And within a short while, a rash of new cases developed. Whereas all the cities that continued with their preventive measures for a long time, never experienced a second wave of high death rates.

So, from the studies carried out in 1918, it was found that the key to reducing the curve was social distancing. And that may likely remain a powerful tool even a century later, in the fight against recent pandemics.

Now in the year 2020, the world is battling on how to curtail the current pandemic that is spreading swiftly across the globe.

Some painful lessons were learned from the 1918 pandemic which are still very relevant today -- and could possibly help to prevent an equally catastrophic outcome.

Chapter Three: Lessons Learnt from the 1918 Spanish Flu

Lesson #1: Don't ease up on social distancing too soon

During the 1918 Spanish flu pandemic, social distancing was stopped too early. And that led to a second wave of infections that was even deadlier than the first, epidemiologists say.

Because of the high rate of fatalities and insufficient spaces in hospitals, the Oakland Municipal Auditorium in California was converted to a makeshift hospital having to employ volunteer nurses from the American Red Cross in 1918.

It is a true fact that there was a large gathering towards the end of the first wave in 1918 which helped to fuel the deadlier second wave.

In San Francisco for example, when the number of Spanish flu cases was almost down to zero, "the city fathers decided to open up the city. They insisted on holding a great big parade downtown. They said: Let's all take off our masks together.

Two months after that event, the influenza came back again and this time it hit very harsh on them.

Also, in the US, the city of Philadelphia suffered a similar circumstance.

Though some 600 sailors from the Philadelphia Navy Yard had contacted the Spanish flu in September of 1918 and came into the city, the city didn't cancel a parade that it scheduled for September 28, 1918.

Three days later, Philadelphia had 635 new cases of the Spanish flu, this was the record gotten from the University of Pennsylvania Archives & Records Center.

And within a very short period Philadelphia was recorded as the city with the highest number of influenza death toll in the US.

Contrasting the above scenario with St. Louis. The city scheduled a similar parade but canceled it and they had a far better record.

The next month after Philadelphia carried out its parade, more than 10,000 people in the city died from the pandemic flu, whereas Saint Louis cases did not go higher than 700, reports from the U.S Centers for Disease Control and Prevention.

We definitely know that different places will reach their different peaks at different times. But note the fact that if one place records less cases with the deadly disease doesn't mean cases or deaths there can't rise again.

Lesson #2: Young, healthy adults can be victims of their strong immune systems

It is important for you to know that the Spanish flu of 1918 killed many young adults that were actually healthy. This was a report given by John M. Barry, a professor at the Tulane University School of Public Health and Tropical Medicine.

There was also a report that about two-thirds of the deaths then were among people between the ages of 18 to 50, "and the peak age for death was 28,". This report was given by Barry, author of "The Great Influenza: The Story of the Deadliest Pandemic in History."

In the years preceding the 1918 flu pandemic, life expectancy in the US was in the early 50s. But a year after the disease struck, the average US life expectancy reduced by 12 years.

When it got to 2017, the average life expectancy in US was 78.6 years. And with the outbreak of this recent pandemic, the elderly and those having underlying health problems are at higher risk for severe complications and possibly death.

Yet a lot of young and healthy adults with strong immune system are dying from the disease.

One major reason why the 1918 flu was so deadly for young adults was because the outbreak started during World War 1. This was the period when many soldiers were in the barracks and they had close proximity with each other. Social distancing could not be implemented in this case.

It was recorded that the United States military training camps had high mortality rate.

Today there isn't any world war, but we have taken a clue and learnt important lessons from the past: young, healthy people are not invincible neither are they immune from the virus. So young adults cannot afford to be careless now, without observing social distancing nor personal hygiene and then rely on their strong immune systems as it might work against them.

The picture above is of flu patients lying in a barracks hospital at Colorado Agricultural College in Fort Collins, Colorado, in 1918.

When scientist of today look back at the Spanish flu, they now believe that there is such a thing as "immune system overreaction, which contributed to the high rate of death among healthy young adults in 1918".

Now a century after the 1918 pandemic has passed. We could also see that a hyperactive immune system can be a contributing factor to young people's deaths from the deadly disease we are currently combating with, says Dr. Sanjay Gupta, a CNN Chief Medical Correspondent. These overly strong responses to the virus are commonly called cytokine storms.

Young and healthy people can have what is called "reactive immune system". And this reactive immune system can result to a chronic inflammatory problem, which can take over the lungs and other organs of the body.

According to Dr. Gupta, he said that "it is not the old or weakened immune system that is the problem, but actually the one that works too well."

Lesson #3: Don't throw unproven drugs at the virus

Actually, we have had some major medical and technological advancement in the past century, like 102 years past. But the Spanish flu and the recent pandemics share two major challenges: the lack of a vaccine and the lack of a cure.

In the 1918 scenario, the remedies provided varied from the newly developed drugs to oils and herbs.

In 2020, there is now a widespread speculation about hydroxychloroquine -- a drug used to treat malaria, lupus and rheumatoid arthritis, whether it could help patients with the recent deadly disease.

The President of America, Donald Trump has made comments about the drug- hydroxychloroquine, when he said, that you don't have anything to lose when by taking the drug. After this statement, some people started to keep the drugs to themselves, even though it's still being tested and has not yet been proven to be a cure to the current pandemic.

A recent research has been carried out and it was found that hydroxychloroquine did not help hospitalized patients with this 2020 deadly disease -- rather, some patients developed abnormal heart rhythms.

With this finding, it is obvious that hydroxychloroquine cannot treat patients with the disease we are now fighting.

From the research also it was discovered that the drug has side effects. It causes heart problems that requires it to be removed from circulation."

Some doctors in Brazil and Sweden have also showed concerns on the use of chloroquine, a drug that is similar to hydroxychloroquine, on patients with this deadly disease because of heart problems.

The conclusion is: It's still not known whether some drugs will cause more harm than good in the fight against the current pandemic.

Chapter Four: Spanish Flu Of 1918 Compared to The Current Pandemic

Although the world at different times had to combat several deadly pandemics over the past century, one of the worst ever recorded was the 1918 influenza pandemic, otherwise called Spanish flu. From studies carried out, it was discovered that the cause of the flu was an H1N1 virus that originated in birds. The first place the flu was identified was in the U.S. in military personnel in the spring of 1918. It got the name "Spanish flu" because there was a speculation that went out at that time that it originated in Spain. But from a research that was published in 2005, it was suggested that the flu actually originated in New York.

One commonality between the Spanish flu's H1N1 and this recent 2020 pandemic is that both are regarded as "novel," that is to say, they are so new nobody in either era had any immunity to them. One striking difference between the two is that those mostly affected in the 1918 pandemic were actually healthy adults between the ages of 20 to 40. The mortality rate was also higher in people younger than five years of age and 65 and older.

"The 1918 pandemic strain influenza was new and one of its kind for most people under the age of 40 or 50, but that's where the death rate really was high—and that's quite different than the usual flu, this report was given by "Mark Schleiss, a pediatric infectious disease specialist at the University of Minnesota told Healthline.

Demographics of the Pandemic

Those mostly affected by this recent disease caused by a deadly virus are actually adults who are above age 65 and having underlying health conditions. From most of the report given, children seem to have not too serious symptoms.

No vaccines were provided for the Spanish flu and there are currently no vaccines for the recent pandemic. A major reason why the Spanish flu was so serious was because there were no antibiotics to treat secondary bacterial infections, so the efforts to control the disease around the globe were limited to non-pharmaceutical responses like isolation, quarantine, disinfectants and reducing public gatherings, although then unlike now, these measures were applied erratically. It was in 1940 that the first flu vaccine to be licensed in the U.S. came on board.

The Spanish flu of 1918 ended in the summer of 1919. Another important fact to take into consideration for the 1918 pandemic was that the world was in the middle of a war and soldiers were spreading the virus globally. Majority of the people also lived in crowded conditions and had extremely poor hygiene.

The current world's population is about 8 billion people with significantly lower death rates from the recent pandemic. Even though the pandemic is not over, the lower figure of affected cases is possibly related to better awareness of how viruses and spread. We would also give credit to better healthcare facilities, both in terms of easy access to hospitals, availability of antibiotics, antiviral drugs and other approaches to treating diseases. Also, though healthcare facilities and hospitals are somewhat overstretched by this current pandemic in many countries, take note that it was quite a bit worse in 1918, as the hospitals then had to deal with mass casualties and injuries from the war, and most of the physicians were with the troops, only medical students were left to take care of the influenza patients.

But today, we have a world that is far more connected with air travel and lesser populations, making the rate of spread of diseases lesser.

Cautions on Comparison

Having looked at the similarities between the past and present pandemic, there are however several significant differences between the two. First difference is that the current pandemic is not influenza. Though they are both caused by novel viruses, but different types of viruses with different methods of action and infectiousness.

Also, global communication and sharing of information have significantly improved, better than in 1918, which has seen researchers sharing data on the pandemic, the virus and numerous drugs, and governments also doing the same.

CONCLUSION/HOPE

The recent pandemic ravaging the world is without a doubt an enormous and unique challenge all over the earth and the battle is nowhere near being over. But there are signs that government policies in several countries, including Germany and South Korea, have been able to contain the virus. Even in China, where the pandemic appears to have originated, seems three months later, to have things largely under control.

As Ross Douthat wrote in The New York Times on March 28, there are signs of what he calls "rational hope," which "is not the same as reckless optimism. It doesn't require, for instance, quickly lifting quarantines based on outlying projections of low fatality rates, as some return-to-normalcy conservatives have been doing in the last week. A rational hope will accept that the situation is actually worse, but then it still looks around for signs leading up and out. It recognizes that things are likely to get worse but keeps itself alert to the contexts in which they seem to be getting better—or at the very least, getting worse more slowly."

As earlier stated, the pandemics, from the 1918 Spanish flu to the H1N1 pandemic of 2009, actually ended. Sometimes with seemingly unbearable numbers of deaths, but eventually they do end.